THE PORTUGUESE COOKBOOK

Traditionally Recipes

Andrea C. Barto

Contents

Chapter 1

INTRODUCTION

In the 15th century, Prince Henry the Navigator instructed his explorers to bring any exotic fruits, nuts, and plants discovered in new lands back to Portugal. As a result, the Age of Discovery had a significant impact on Portuguese and international cooking.

Brazilian pineapples were introduced to the Azores, Brazilian chili peppers thrived in Angola, African coffee was transplanted to Brazil (which now produces roughly half of the world's supply), Brazilian cashews were introduced to Africa and India, and Europeans were introduced to tea. Spices such as cinnamon and curry powder, for example, are still popular in Portugal today as a result of this period. Other cultures, on the other hand, had been bringing new foods to Portugal for centuries. In order to make the Iberian Peninsula the granary of Rome, the Romans transported wheat and introduced onions, garlic, olives, and grapes to it. Later, throughout the Algarve province, the Moors were the first to cultivate rice, introduce figs, plant lemon and orange groves, and plant almond trees.

Naturally, modern Portuguese cuisine varies by region, but fresh fish and shellfish appear on nearly every menu. The national dish is Bacalhau (dried, salted cod). The Portuguese have had a fascination with Newfoundland since their fishing boats arrived there in the early 16th century. The sailors salted and sun-dried their catch to make it last the long journey home, and there are now 365 ways to prepare it, one for each day of the year, according to legend.

Roasted sardines and horse mackerel, as well as a stew made with a variety of fish known as "Caldeirada," are also popular in coastal communities.

Across the country, specialty seafood restaurants abound, with many of them displaying lobsters, shrimp, oysters, and crabs in inventive ways. To sample a combination of them, order the rich seafood rice "arroz de marisco."

Another national cuisine is "cozido à portuguesa," a thick stew of vegetables with a variety of meats. The most common type is pork, which can be prepared and consumed in a variety of ways. Roast suckling pig ("leito assado") and pork sausages known as "chouriço" or "linguiça" are popular in the north of the country.

A typical Porto dish is tripe with haricot beans. It isn't for everyone, but it has been Porto's most famous dish since Henry the Navigator dispatched a ship to conquer Ceuta in Morocco, and the residents of Porto slaughtered all their livestock to feed the crew, keeping only the intestines for themselves. They've been known as "tripeiros" or "tripe eaters" since then.

Breakfast is usually just coffee and a bread roll, but lunch is a substantial meal that can take up to two hours to complete. Dinner is usually served after 8:00 p.m., between noon and 2:00 p.m., or between 1:00 and 2:00 p.m. Soup is a popular addition to the three-course meal. The most popular soup is cado verde, which contains potato, chopped kale, and sausage bits.

Cinnamon-flavored rice pudding, flan, and caramel custard are the most popular desserts, but there are also a variety of cheeses available. The most popular variations use sheep or goat's milk, with "queijo da serra" from the Serra da Estrela region being the most popular.

In the 18th century, nuns made many of the country's most beautiful pastries, which they sold to supplement their income. "Barriga de Freira" ("nun's belly"), "papos de anjo" ("angel's chests"), and "toucinho do céu" ("toucinho of the sky") are just a few of the imaginative titles ("bacon from heaven"). The "pastel de nata," a small custard tart dusted with cinnamon, is one of the most delicious pastries.

Enjoy the bread on the table before any meal in a restaurant in Lisbon or anywhere else in Portugal. Portugal's bread is exceptional.

Chapter 2

PORTUGUESE CUISINE UNDERSTANDING

With our comprehensive reference to Portuguese cuisine, you can learn about the many flavors and culinary traditions of the sunny Iberian Peninsula.

If you enjoy seafood and a Mediterranean diet, you'll love Portugal's growing culinary scene. Aside from fish, you can expect to find a wide variety of regional delicacies. This includes everything from rich cheeses and unusual bread to smoky sausages and sweet desserts, all of which are accompanied by excellent Port.

To give you an idea of the culinary delights in store, this Portuguese food guide includes the following information:

A culinary tour of Portugal Diet in Portugal

Portuguese cuisine is divided into regions. Pantry of Portugal

Easy Substitutes in the Modern Culinary Scene

PORTUGUESE CUISINE IN CONTEXT

In 1279, King Diniz invested in the development of Portugal's naval forces, marking the start of the country's involvement in world exploration and colonialism. By the late 1300s, Portuguese marine captains were among Europe's best, having completed numerous missions with great success. It was Italy that was the first European country to dock in Japan, China, and Ethiopia, bringing with them a plethora of new and exotic goods. As a result, the Portuguese contributed significantly to food globalization. They brought Asian rice, tea, and peanuts from Africa, as well as pineapples, peppers, tomatoes, and potatoes from the New World. Also brought to Europe by the Portuguese were coriander, pepper, ginger, curry, saffron, and paprika.

Because of the country's long and rich history of colonization, Portuguese influences can be found in cuisines all over the world. Brazilian cuisine, for example, has its own adaptations of Portuguese dishes, as do regional delicacies in Macau and

Goa. The country is also credited with bringing grain to Africa. In the 1660s, tea became fashionable in England after the Portuguese princess Catherine of Braganza brought her taste for Macau leaves to the English court.

In recent years, Portugal has faced economic inequity, which has resulted in health and nutritional problems. Indeed, the World Health Organization (WHO) discovered that consuming more trans fatty acids, sugar, and salt has increased obesity, diabetes, and malnutrition rates in the country. As a result, the Portuguese government is promoting healthier food and beverage alternatives. Despite this, according to the most recent Global Nutrition Report, Portugal has a long way to go in terms of being a healthy country.

THE DIET OF THE PORTUGUESE

Portugal's cuisine is mostly based on hearty peasant meals and a Mediterranean lifestyle. Seafood lovers will definitely appreciate the effect of the country's huge Atlantic coastline on traditional cuisine. The tastes and ingredients differ depending on where in Portugal you are.

Breakfast

In Portugal, breakfast is referred to as pequeno almoço, which translates to'small lunch.' This is often drunk before 9:00 a.m. It's a little lunch made out of fresh bread, butter, ham, and cheese or jam, as the name suggests. For breakfast, people also consume cereal with milk or yogurt and fruit. The most typical morning drinks are coffee, milk, and tea.

Breakfast is also quite popular in Portugal, particularly the freshly baked pastel de nata, which is a national dish. These are best served with a shot of espresso in the morning or as an afternoon snack.

Lunch

Lunch (almoço) is given much more attention in Portugal, and it frequently lasts more than an hour, between 12:00 and 14:00. Even though it is eaten at work, lunch is a social occasion. Lunch and dinner in Portugal normally consist of three major dishes, including soup. Green broth (caldo verde) is a traditional Portuguese soup prepared with pureed potatoes, onions, and garlic.

After that, the collard greens are shredded and mixed in. Despite the fact that the dish may be made vegetarian, chouriço slices are usually served with it (a smoked or spicy Portuguese sausage).

Dinner

You'll be thankful for your lengthy, substantial lunch while you wait for supper in Portugal. Dinner (jantar) is usually served between 20:00 and 21:00, or even later on weekends. As previously indicated, it usually consists of three courses and includes soup.

Soups are often served as the main course. One of these soups is sopa de marisco, or shellfish soup with wine.

Caldeirada, a fish stew made with a variety of species, and carne de porco an Alentejana, pork wrapped in clam and tomato sauce, are two more Portuguese specialities. Despite the fact that most major meals in Portugal involve meat or fish, peixinhos da horta is a popular vegetarian dish.

Snacks

Anyone who likes grazing all day would love Lanche in Portugal. It literally means'snack,' despite its similarities to the phrase lunch. Snacking is common in Portugal between breakfast and lunch. You may not have had your daily pastel de nata yet, for example.

DIFFERENCES IN PORTUGUESE CUISINE BY REGION

Despite the fact that Portugal is a small nation, its food reflects diverse regional influences. As a consequence, where you reside in the nation will have a big impact on the food you consume.

Northern Portugal and the city of Porto

The country's northern areas are known for their hearty, robust cuisine. In the upper right corner, the area of Trás-os-Montes proudly claims to be the origin of feijoada. In Portugal, this bean stew has grown highly popular. Also available is alheira, a smoked sausage made with poultry, bread, and fat. Arroz de cabidela, on the other hand, is a rice dish prepared with chicken or game cooked in its own blood.

Tripe dishes are prominent in the city, notably the well-known tripas à moda do Porto. Naturally, Port wine is produced in the Alto Douro Valley Wine Region in northern Portugal. Vinho Verde wines are also made in the north.

Portugal's central region

The Aveiro estuary in central Portugal is regarded to have the country's best oysters. A lot of game meat may be found on restaurants all across the area. A typical delicacy is Pastel de Molho da Covilh, a filo pastry filled with ground pig cooked with onions and bay leaves. Another local cuisine is bucho, a flavorful combination of rice and pork meat cooked inside a pig's stomach. Caldeirada à Ria de Aveiro, a regional fish stew with pork and ginger powder, is also popular.

Alejento

Alejento dishes often include lamb or pig, although trout is also popular. Another regional speciality is B bread and bean broth soup, which is ideal for dipping Alentejo bread in. Because it is typical in Alentejo, the round and compact form of the native Evora cheese is also instantly recognizable. This somewhat yellow cheese comes in three different textures: ripened, hard, and semi-hard. With eight subregions producing wine, Alentejo is one of Portugal's top wine regions.

Chapter 3

THE PANTRY OF PORTUGAL

Lisbon

In Lisbon, which sits on an estuary near the ocean, fish and seafood are always on the menu. Since the Moors conquered the city in the early eighth century, sardines have been a staple of the local cuisine. You may now purchase nicely adorned sardine jars in cafés and bars and consume canned sardines (conservas) with numerous garnishes.

Some of Portugal's most well-known recipes originate in Lisbon. The pastel de nata (custard tart) is supposed to have been developed in Lisbon's majestic Monasterio de Jerónimos in Belém, right next to a sugar cane factory. The national dish, bacalhau com broa, is also made in Lisbon (cod baked with cornmeal).

Portugal's south

Shellfish abound in the cuisine of the Algarve. Conquilhas à Algarvia, for example, is a clam dish with fried onions, garlic, and chopped Portuguese sausage. There are other pastries containing sweet marzipan or figs. In the Algarve, these doces finos, which are shaped into diverse forms, are a source of considerable cultural pride. In seafood meals in the Montanhas area, you'll mostly find eel or trout. The main draws here are alheiras, veal sausages, chicken, and ham.

I've stocked portions of my pantry and refrigerator with goods that I use in my kitchen to cook Portuguese dishes. Through trial and error, I've discovered American ingredients that are either similar to or successful substitutes for those found in Portugal. Nothing irritates me more than thinking one thing when an author means another, so in these entries, I've stated the precise onion variety, bay leaf kind, and ideal potato cultivar to use in making the recipes in the United States, so that we're all on the same page. It's not an exhaustive list; it just covers the items needed to make the recipes in this book. Some of the more difficult-to-find foods, such as Portuguese sausages and bottled sauces, are listed below.

The most important factor in the success of your cuisine is, without a doubt, purchasing the highest-quality ingredients you can afford. Conjure up the guts to ask your fishmonger about salt cod, then skip the discount bin and spend on a well-priced sumptuous port wine you wouldn't mind enjoying after an incredible time cooking by gently poking a few tomatoes in the name of price matching.

Oh, and I've added a small pronunciation instruction since Portuguese is tough to speak. Best of luck!

BACON toucinho (in Portuguese) (tow-seen-yoo)

Pork is the king of meat in Portugal, and nose-to-tail eating is the custom. Authors and interpreters of Portuguese recipes, on the other hand, have left chefs banging their heads against kitchen cabinets for years by indiscriminately using the word bacon to refer to toucinho. Toucinho is available in three varieties, one of which is similar to bacon as we know it, and each has its own cooking application.

Toucinho gordo ("fat bacon") is 100% pork fat, similar to our fatback, with no meat striations and often intact skin. It may be cut from almost any section of the animal and is normally salted (salgado) rather than smoked, however smoked toucinho magro and toucinho entremeado are also available. Chunks are used in dishes such as feijoada (bean-meat casserole), cozido (a one-pot meal of cooked meats and vegetables), and even desserts.

The meat-to-fat ratio of Toucinho magro ("thin bacon") is greater. This kind of toucinho was originally chunked, fried until crisp, and preserved in a clay pot until ready to use in meals. These recipes don't call for this type of bacon, but if you come across extremely lean farmhouse bacon, try it.

Toucinho entremeado is a smoked, not salted, half-fat, half-meat toucinho entremeado. This bacon is the most similar to ours, and it's what I used to develop the recipes in this book. To get the same flavor, use slab bacon or pancetta instead of boxed sliced bacon, even if it isn't smoked. At all costs, stay away from flavored bacons like maple or mesquite.

Chapter 4

HOW TO MAKE RICE

B

DESSERTS

CUSTARD TARTS

Makes 24 tarts

Ingredients\sPASTRY

275 g (10 oz/2¼ cups) plain (all-purpose) flour, plus more to dust

¼ teaspoon fine salt

125–175 ml (4–6 fl oz/½–¾ cup) chilled water

200 g (7 oz) (7 oz) unsalted butter, beaten till the time soft, nonetheless not melted

CUSTARD FILLING

250 g (9 oz/1¼ cups) caster (superfine) (superfine) sugar 150 ml (5 fl oz/ ⅔ cup) water\s600 ml (1 pint/2½ cups) whole milk 1 vanilla pod, split lengthways

½ cinnamon stick\spared rind of ½ unwaxed lemon, slice into long strips 12 egg yolks\sicing (confectioners') sugar, in order to serve ground cinnamon, in order to serve

Directions

Using a spoon and then your hands, blend combining the flour, salt and as much chilled water as necessary in a vesssel to prepare a soft, light dough. The moment it begins to come together, turn it out of the vesssel and onto a floured work surface. Press then roll it out to make a 15 cm (6 in) square. Wrap the pastry in plastic wrap and chill in the refrigerator for twenty minutes. Roll out the chilled pastry to make a rough 45 cm (18 in) square, with the help of lots of flour to avoid it sticking to the surface or the rolling pin. Trim to make a neat square. Divide the soft butter into three coarsely equal quantities. In case it is looking shimmering or beginning to melt, pautilize here and chill it and the pastry for ten minutes. Utilize a palette knife or spatula to spread one third of the butter over the left-hand two thirds of the pastry, leaving a 3 cm (1¼ in) gap all around the edge. Working swiftly, fold the un-buttered right-hand third over the buttered centre third. (Utilize a pastry scraper or palette knife to loosen the dough, in case needed.) Working from the top down, dab the pastry to get rid of any air bubbles. Touch the pastry as less as possible, to prevent it getting as well warm. Now, fold the buttered left-hand third over as well, so that it covers newly visible un- buttered pastry. You must have access to a long rectangle of pastry and no visible butter. Pat for a short time to get rid of any bubbles. At this stage, the butter within the pastry layers can turn a bit soft, particularly on a hot day. In case this happens, chill the dough for ten minutes to allow the butter to firm up.

Makes 12 doughnuts

Ingredients

DOUGHNUTS

1 tablespoon active dry yeast 150 ml (5 fl oz/ ⅔ cup) to some extent warm whole milk

50 g (2 oz/¼ cup) caster (superfine) sugar, plus three-four tablespoons for coating the doughnuts 50 g (2 oz) salted butter, melted and cooled

2 eggs, plus 1 yolk pinch of salt

500 g (1 lb 2 oz/four cups) plain (all-purpose) flour, plus extra to dust flavourless oil, for greasing vesssel and for frying

FILLING

250 ml (8½ fl oz/1 cup) whole milk 1 teaspoon vanilla extract ½ cinnamon stick

2 pared strips of unwaxed lemon zest 50 g (2 oz/¼ cup) caster (superfine) sugar four egg yolks

1 tablespoon plain (all-purpose) flour 1½ tablespoons cornflour

Directions

Mix the yeast with the just-warm milk and sugar in a jug or a container to activate it.

Allow for a ten-minute rest period, during which time it should form a frothy head.

Melt and whisk the cooled melted butter, eggs and yolks, and salt together, then meld and mix the egg mixture into the yeasty milk once the yeast has done its thing.

Make a well in the center of the flour in a large mixing bowl, then pour in the milk–egg mixture. Stir with a wooden spoon, then use your hands to bring it together into a rough ball once it starts to form a dough. Turn it out onto a floured surface and knead for about ten minutes with floured hands, adding a little more flour if it's too sticky, until the dough is smooth and elastic. Alternatively, knead the dough for six minutes in a stand blender fitted with a dough hook. Place the smooth, soft dough in a clean, lightly oiled vesssel, cover with plastic wrap, and set aside to rise for one hour or more, or until it has doubled in size. Prepare the filling while you wait. Allow to come to a boil in a saucepan with the milk, vanilla extract, cinnamon stick, and strips of lemon zest, then remove from the heat. In a heavy vesssel, melt and combine the sugar, egg yolks, and both flours until smooth and creamy. Remove the cinnamon and lemon zest from the milk, as well as any surface skin. Whisk vigorously 1 tablespoon hot milk into the egg yolk mixture. Continue to add a tablespoon of hot milk at a time, whisking quickly to prevent the eggs from cooking and scrambling. (Using a heavy vessel will keep it from moving while whisking with one hand and decanting with the other.) Decant the mixture into the saucepan in a steady stream, whisking the entire time, after adding 6–7 tablespoons of milk. To prevent lumps from forming, make sure to get into the corners of the pan. Place the saucepan over the lowest heat possible and cook, whisking constantly, for five to ten minutes, until the custard thickens. Remove the pan from the heat and whisk for another three to four minutes. Even more thickening of the custard is required. To prevent a skin from forming, pour the custard into a heat-resistant container and cover the surface with plastic wrap. Allow to cool, then chill for at least one hour in the refrigerator to firm up before using. Turn the dough out of the vesssel and knock it back to its original size before cutting it into 12 equal-sized pieces. Each piece should be rolled into a tight ball and placed on a floured baking sheet. Allow for another thirty minutes of resting in a warm place. Fill a deep frying pan with about 6 cm (212 in) of flavorless oil and place it over a high flame when you're ready to cook. Heat the oil until it reaches 160°C (320°F) on a thermometer – any hotter and the doughnuts will brown quickly but remain raw in the center. Cook 2–3 doughnuts at a time in the heated oil for two and a half to three minutes on each side, or until golden brown on the outside and fluffy and fully cooked inside. (You may need to sacrifice one of your first batch to determine if it is fully cooked.) Using a paper towel-lined platter, drain the fish. Roll the hot doughnuts in the remaining three-four tablespoons of caster sugar in a shallow dish. Cut each one in half with a sharp knife, then fill with a heaping tablespoonful or two of the chilled, firm custard, like a sandwich. Serve right away – they won't last long, and you won't want them to!

DOUGHNUTS THAT ARE VERY LONG

There are about 15 doughnuts in this recipe.

Ingredients

812 fl oz (1 cup) 250 ml water

salted butter, 3 tblsp salt, a pinch

5 oz/114 cups = 150 g merely flour 3 eggs, beaten\sflavourless oil, for frying

½ teaspoon ground cinnamon

5 tablespoons caster (superfine) (superfine) sugar

Directions

Bring the water, butter and salt to the boil in a non-stick saucepan over a medium–high flame. The moment the butter has melted, put in the flour, all simultaneously. Turn down the flame to low and blend rapidly with a wooden spoon: the blend will appear lumpy and terrible, nonetheless will turn into a soft dough that pulls away from the sides of the pan. Cook over a low flame for three minutes. Place the dough moving, with the help of the spoon to massage the ball of dough so that the heat is uniformly distributed. Now, put the dough in the vesssel of a stand blender fitted with a paddle attachment and beat till the time it is optimally cool to touch. Put in the eggs, a bit of at a time, with the blender running. You may not require them all, and each time you add some egg, the blend will appear as though it's approximately to split, nonetheless keep beating. The dough is done when it is soft, light and elastic. As another option, beat the eggs in by hand. Put a wide, deep saucepan over a high flame and fill it with four cm (1½ in) of the flavourless oil. Heat the oil till the time it reaches 170°C (340°F) on a saucepan thermometer, or in case you don't have one, utilize the bread test: once the oil is gleaming, drop in a cube of day-old bread. In case the bread fizzes and browns in no less than thirty seconds, the oil is done. (In case it burns in that time, turn down the flame.) Scoop the dough into a piping bag fitted with a large nozzle

(In case you don't have one, don't worry, just spoon little balls of the dough into the oil). Cautiously pipe thick sausages of dough directly into the warmed up oil, pinching them off the moment they reach your desired length – which can be anything from 6–15 cm (2½–6 in) long. Don't crowd the saucepan as that will cautilize the oil temperature to put and make the doughnuts flabby and greasy. Cook for 5–six minutes, turning them once or twice, till the time puffed up, crispy and a deep golden brown. The doughnuts can every now and then spit, so it's utilizeful to have splatter guard to rest on top of the saucepan in case of oily splashes. Remove the farturas as you draw them out of the oil and onto a platter lined with paper towel. Blend the sugar and cinnamon together in a shallow vesssel and when optimally

cool to touch, roll the doughnuts in it. Doughnuts don't keep well, so Consume while warm, with coffee or hot chocolate.

MERINGUE CLOUDS WITH CUSTARD

Serves 6–8

Ingredients\s750 ml (25 fl oz/3 cups) whole milk 1 cinnamon stick\spared rind of 1 unwaxed lemon, slice into long strips, plus not many drops of its juice four eggs, always at room temperature pinch of salt

200 g (7 oz/scant 1 cup) caster (superfine) sugar

1 tablespoon cornflour\sdash of cold milk (optional)
(optional)

ground cinnamon, in order to serve (optional) (optional)

Directions

Put a large, wide saucepan over a low hconsume, and put in
the milk, accompanied by the cinnamon stick and long strips
of lemon rind. Slowly bring the milk to the boil. In the
meantime, separate the whites from the egg yolks very
cautiously, not letting any yolk to get into the whites. Place
the yolks aside. Meld and mix the egg whites with not many
drops of lemon juice and the salt in a spotlessly clean vesssel
till the time they form firm peaks, then add a tablespoon of
the sugar, whisk again, then add another tablespoon.
Replicate with a third tablespoon of sugar. The whites require
to be really firm, or else they will lose their shape during
cooking. Once the milk is boiling, lower the flame to low and
take out the cinnamon stick and strips of lemon rind. Skim
off any skin that has formed on the surface. Utilize 2 large
metal spoons to shape the meringues into large quenelles

(you can dip the spoons in hot water first, in case you wish, to make it easier to shape the blend): hold one spoon in each hand and take a spoonful of the egg white blend with one spoon. Utilize the other spoon to lightly shape and rotate the meringue, turning it lightly till the time it is sitting on that spoon; replicate a number of times till the time the meringue is a fairly smooth oblong, then slide it into the milk. Reliant on the size of your pan, replicate once or twice, till the time you have 2–3 meringues floating in the milk. Allow the meringues to cook for approximately one minute, then lightly turn them over in the milk to cook for another minute – don't worry in case little bits of the meringue fall off into the milk. Take out the cooked meringues using a slotted spoon and put aside to drain in a large colander, or on a plate. Get rid of any more skin which has formed on the milk and replicate the process till the time all the meringue blend has been utilized up. Take out the milk from the heat. To make the custard, blend combining the cornflour and rest of the sugar in a heavy vesssel, then put in the egg yolks and beat till the time smooth. Add a ladleful of the hot milk, whisk coarsely, and replicate a number of times, whisking uninterruptedly. (Using a heavy vesssel will stop the vesssel moving as you whisk with one hand and decant with

the other.) Pass the remaining hot milk through a sieve into a clean saucepan and gradually decant in the egg yolk blend, whisking uninterruptedly. Transfer the saucepan over medium flame and allow to come to a simmer, mixing constantly. The moment the custard starts to thicken (after five-ten minutes), take out the saucepan from the hconsume, nonetheless continue to stir for five minutes or so. It should be a decanting consistency – in case the custard seems as well thick, add a bit of cold milk. Draw the drained meringues from the colander or plate, leaving any liquid behind, and add in serving dish. Spoon over some of the custard, and dust with cinnamon, in case required.

SWEETENED EGG YOLKS Ingredients 8 egg yolks 250 g (9 oz/1¼ cups) caster (superfine) sugar 150 ml (5 fl oz/ ⅔ cup) water

Directions

Meld and mix the egg yolks in a heavy mixing vesssel till the time smooth and creamy.

Put a deep saucepan over a high flame and put in the sugar and water. Heat the blend till the time it reaches 105°C (221°F) on a saucepan thermometer. Take off of the flame and let rest to cool for a number of minutes. Decant the syrup, very slowly, into the egg yolks, beating uninterruptedly with a whisk. (Using a heavy vessel will keep it from moving while whisking with one hand and decanting with the other.) Once all the syrup has been added to the yolks, decant the egg yolk syrup back into the pan. Place over a very low flame and cook, mixing, for 5–six minutes, till the time it has thickened – it should appear like a bright yellow or orange custard. (Don't let the blend get as well hot or boil, as it will split and become grainy.) Take out the saucepan from the heat and leave the custard to cool. It will keep in the refrigerator for not many days. Utilize to top or fill cakes or pastries, like the Santa Clara Pastries mentioned. QUINCE & PORT WINE BAKED APPLES

Serves 4

Ingredients

four medium-sized cooking apples, cored nonetheless unpeeled four tablespoons quince paste or quince cheese

four tablespoons light muscovado sugar, plus more for sprinkling four tablespoons port wine

¼ teaspoon ground cinnamon

four teaspoons salted butter, plus extra to grease creamy vanilla ice cream, or custard, in order to serve

Directions

Heat beforehand the oven to 180°C (350°F/Gas 4).

Score a line around the circumference of each apple, using a sharp knife, just deep sufficient to break the skin.

Grease a baking dish, and transfer the apples into it, sitting them on their bases. Blend combining the quince paste, sugar, port and cinnamon in a vesssel. Utilize your fingers to poke this blend into the holes where the cores were, dividing the blend equally between the apples. Top each hole with a teaspoon of butter and drizzle over a tad bit more sugar. Once all the apples are filled and have been drizzled with the extra sugar, decant sufficient water into the dish to reach approximately 1 cm (½ in) up the sides of the apples. Add in the preheated oven and cook for 35–45 minutes, till the time the apples are entirely cooked through. Serve alongside the syrupy juices from the baking dish and some creamy vanilla ice cream or custard. FRESH CHEESE WITH FIGS

Serves 4

Ingredients 12 fresh, ripe green or purple figs 75 g (2½ oz/¾ cup) flaked almonds

200 g (7 oz) Queijo Fresco Cheese or other fresh mild cheese such as ricotta 2 tablespoons honey

Directions

Halve each of the figs, or in case they're very plump, quarter them. Set on a platter or in a large serving dish. Transfer the almonds into a dry frying saucepan set over medium flame and toast lightly till the time light gold in colour. Tear or crumble the cheese into large pieces and distribute it over the figs, followed by the toasted almonds. Lastly, sprinkle the honey over, and serve instantly. FLOURLESS CHOCOLATE CAKES WITH LIME CREAM

Makes 12 cakes

Ingredients 200 g (7 oz) good-quality dark chocolate (70 percent cocoa solids minimum), broken into chunks 200 g (7 oz) salted butter, plus extra to grease

four eggs

100 g (3½ oz/½ cup) raw cane sugar or soft brown sugar 1 tablespoon very strong black coffee

2 tablespoons aged rum 200 ml (7 fl oz/generous ¾ cup) whipping cream grated zest of ½ lime

12 teaspoons Dulce de Leche

Directions

Heat beforehand the oven to 180°C (350°F/Gas 4) and grease a 12-hole muffin tin with butter.

Heat the chocolate and butter in a bain-marie or a heat resistant vesssel set over a saucepan of just-simmering water, till the time melted and shiny (don't allow the vesssel to touch the water or the chocolate will overheat). Take off of the flame and let rest to cool to some extent. Meld and mix the eggs, sugar, coffee and rum together in a vesssel for three-four minutes, till the time pale brown and moussy – the beaters should leave trails across the surface of the blend when lifted up. Utilize a large metal spoon or plastic spatula to fold together the chocolate blend and the egg blend, employing a swiping motion through the blend instead of stirring. This may feel like it's taking ages nonetheless it's the best method to avoid knocking all the precious air out of the eggs. Decant the blend into the holes of the greased muffin tin, nonetheless don't fill to the top; leave 2 mm (⅛ in) or so for the puddings to rise, or they will spill over. Take the tin into the oven and bake for 1three minutes, or till the time the cakes have puffed up proudly. Take off of the oven and cool completely, in the tin. As they cool, the middle of the cakes will sink (this is normal). Lightly turn the cakes out of the tin, running a palette knife or spatula around the edges to loosen in case needed. Whip the cream in a vesssel till the time it forms soft peaks, then stir in the lime zest. Just prior to serving, put a teaspoonful of dulce de leche into the little wells which have formed in the middle of each cake, then top each one with a dollop of the zesty cream. Serve instantly.

CHICKPEA TARTS

Makes 20 tarts

Ingredients butter, to grease

400 g (14 oz) tin chickpeas (garbanzo beans), drained and rinsed (about 230g/8 oz drained weight) 200 g (7 oz/scant 1 cup) caster (superfine) sugar

four egg yolks

½ teaspoon ground cinnamon grated zest of 1 unwaxed lemon

350 g (12 oz) block of all-butter puff pastry dough plain (all-purpose) flour to dust icing (confectioners') sugar, in order to serve (optional)

Directions

Heat beforehand the oven to 180°C (350°F/Gas 4) and grease 1–2 muffin or tart tins with butter.

In an electronic blender, blitz together the chickpeas, sugar, egg yolks, cinnamon and lemon zest till the time smooth.

Bring the pastry to room temperature, then roll it out on a clean, floured surface, with a floured rolling pin and floured hands, till the time it is approximately 3 mm (⅛ in) thick. Cut 20 discs using an 8 cm (3 in) cutter and press them into the greased holes of the tin(s), re-rolling the scraps in case needed (the tarts you roll last might rise a bit unevenly, though). Fill each tart two-thirds full with the chickpea blend, then add into the preheated oven. Cook for twenty to twenty-five minutes, or till the time the pastry is crisp and the filling has puffed up and set on top. Take off of the oven and dust with icing sugar, in case required.

In case you want to make them in advance, they will keep for up to twenty-four hours.

BACON FROM HEAVEN WITH PORT- POACHED PEARS Serves 8

Ingredients CAKE

150 ml (5 fl oz/ ⅔ cup) water

1 tablespoon lard (or butter), plus extra to grease 300 g (10 ½ oz/1½ cups) caster (superfine) sugar pinch of salt

250 g (8 oz/2½ cups) ground almonds (almond meal)

¼ teaspoon ground cinnamon grated zest of ½ unwaxed lemon grated zest of ¼ orange

3 eggs

2 egg yolks icing (confectioners') sugar, in order to serve

PEARS

200 ml (7 fl oz/generous ¾ cup) water 500 ml (17 fl oz/2¼ cups) port wine (choose something cheap) 100 g (3½ oz/scant ½ cup) caster (superfine) sugar

½ cinnamon stick

6 cm (2½ in) strip of orange zest 6 cm (2½ in) strip of unwaxed lemon zest 2 pears vanilla ice cream, or crème fraîche, in order to serve (optional)

Directions

First, make the cake. Heat beforehand the oven to 180°C (350°F/Gas 4) and grease and line the base and sides of a 20 cm (8 in) round cake tin, ideally one with a loose base. Transfer the water, lard, sugar and salt in a large saucepan. allow to come to a boil and cook till the time all the constituents have melted or dissolved in the water. Lower the flame to low, put in the ground almonds and cook, mixing, for approximately five minutes, to allow the almonds to absorb some of the liquid and for the almond paste to thicken. Take off of the flame, stir in the cinnamon and citrus zests, and let rest to cool to some extent. Once the blend has cooled a bit of, beat the eggs and yolks in a vesssel, then add them to the almond paste, mixing well to incorporate. Decant the batter into the prepared cake tin and add in the oven. Bake for 30–35 minutes, till the time golden brown on top. Let rest to cool in the tin and, once lukewarm, invert the cake. Dust with a bit of icing sugar.

Prepare the pears while the cake is cooking or cooling. In a non-reactive saucepan, combine the water, port, sugar, cinnamon stick, and strips of zest and bring to a simmer over medium heat, stirring to dissolve the sugar. Pears should be peeled, quartered, and cored before being sliced into 8 portions. Reduce the heat under the saucepan to a low simmer, then add the pear pieces and poach for 15 to 20 minutes (do not stir, since the fruit will become rather delicate). The pears will be mushy but retain their form after cooking and will have developed a rich maroon color. Remove them from the poaching liquid. Allow to cool after straining. Serve the pears beside the cake, with a scoop of vanilla ice cream or a dollop of crème fraîche on the side.

PUDDING WITH RICE

4 servings

100 g (312 oz/generous 12 cup) of ingredients 650 mL (22 fl oz/234 cups) rice pudding 12 unwaxed lemon zest, peeled and sliced into long strips water sprinkle of salt

12 tsp cinnamon

812 fl oz (1 cup) 250 ml 40 g whole milk (112 oz/scant 14 cup) the caster (superfine) 2 egg yolks, sugar

1 tablespoon butter (ground cinnamon) for serving

Directions

Cook, uncovered, for roughly thirty minutes, until most of the water has drained and the rice is just soft enough in a pot with the water, salt, strips of lemon zest, and cinnamon stick over a low heat.

Heat the milk and sugar in a separate pan after the rice has been cooking for 25 minutes.

In a mixing bowl, whisk the egg yolks until smooth and creamy.

After thirty minutes, reduce the heat under the rice to the lowest level possible and begin to integrate the hot milk-and-sugar mixture into the cooked rice by adding it gently and often, mixing after each addition, similar to risotto. When everything is combined, the rice should have the consistency of thick porridge. Extinguish the flame. To temper the yolks, add a tablespoon of the hot rice mixture to the beaten yolks and incorporate quickly. Then, while still in the pot but off the heat, slowly incorporate the egg-yolk mixture into the remaining rice, mixing quickly. Return the saucepan to a very low heat, add the butter, and simmer for three minutes, stirring constantly to avoid the egg in the bottom of the pan from overheating and splitting.

Serve warm or cold, with cinnamon sprinkled over top, in four serving dishes.

BISCUITS FROM A CAT'S TONGUE

This recipe makes around 20 biscuits.

75 g (212 oz) of ingredients 100 g soft salted butter (312 oz/scant 12 cup) the caster (superfine) 12 teaspoon vanilla extract sugar 2 beaten egg whites

312 oz/34 cup 100 g merely (all-purpose) to grease with flour and flavorless oil (optional)

Directions

Preheat the oven to 200°C (400°F/Gas 6) in advance.

Cream the butter and sugar together in a stand mixer equipped with a beater attachment until light and creamy, then add the vanilla extract and egg whites, mixing briefly to incorporate. Finally, fold in the flour with a metal spoon or a spatula, swiping a swiping motion through the mixture until just incorporated — don't over-mix. Make the biscuit mix by hand if you choose. Use a silicone baking pan to cook these cookies if you have one, since they stick quickly. If not, gently coat a large non-stick baking sheet with oil. Fill a piping bag with the biscuit mixture and pipe 6 2 cm (212 34 in) pieces of the mixture onto the sheet, allowing at least 5 cm (2 in) between each one from side to side and around 3 cm (114 in) from top to bottom, since the biscuits will spread out a lot in the oven. Place in the oven for 8–10 minutes, or until the edges of the biscuits are golden brown (the centres may remain fairly pale). Remove the biscuits from the oven and use a palette knife or spatula to draw them onto a wire rack or dish to cool and firm up while still hot.

In a vacuum container, the biscuits will last for many days.

6 Servings Sweet Rice Pudding

14 teaspoon salt 14 teaspoon kosher salt 14 teaspoon kosher salt 14 teaspoon kosher salt 2 c. liquid

1 cup Italian sticky rice, big chunks of raw lemon rind

1 cinnamon stick

four and a half cups full milk (14 cup used with the egg yolks) four beaten egg yolks

1 teaspoon vanilla extract

14 cup butter (distributed)

Directions

Combine the water and salt in a pan.

Bring to a boil, then add the rice and stir to combine.

Reduce the heat to low and continue to cook, stirring often, until the rice has absorbed the majority of the liquid (about twenty minutes). Allowing it to totally dry out will cause it to burn. In a large mixing bowl, combine the lemon rind, half of the butter, the cinnamon stick, and four cups of milk. Raise the temperature to medium-high. Allow to return to a boil, stirring often, and then reduce to a low burner. Check for any rice that has adhered to the pan's bottom. Cooking time is 20 minutes. Add the remaining butter and continue to stir while boiling for about ten minutes. In a small vessel, whisk together the eggs and 14 cup milk. Pour the egg mixture into the remaining ingredients and simmer for a few minutes more, until the mixture thickens.

Remove the pan from the heat and stir in the vanilla extract.

Remove the lemon rinds and cinnamon stick and discard.

Pour onto a serving dish and season with a pinch of cinnamon on top.

Serve cold or at room temperature at all times. Serve and have fun! Doughnuts de Portugal (serves 20)

1 tbsp yeast 1 tbsp sugar 1 tbs

6 eggs, room temperature at all times

a third of a cup of warm water, split into two 12 pound portions flour for baking

14 cup milk 12 teaspoon salt tablespoons vegetable shortening four tablespoons sugar, divided

a third of a cup of water, oil for frying, and sugar for sprinkling

Directions

In a 14 cup of warm water, dissolve your yeast and 1 teaspoon of sugar, then set away.

Beat your eggs with 1 spoonful of sugar in a vesssel until they achieve a thick consistency.

Melt the butter in a saucepan, then add the milk, shortening, and the remaining heated water. Allow to cool to a certain level.

While mixing, decant in the egg yolks.

Combine the flour and salt in a mixing bowl.

Pour in the egg mixture and mix with your fingertips.

Half of the water is added, and the mixture is folded in half from the edges to the middle. Repeat as needed.

Knead in your yeast mixture and continue to knead.

Gradually add additional water to the vesssel, making the dough moist and sticky.

Continue to knead the dough until it begins to stay together.

Take a portion the size of an egg and stretch it out to test whether it can be stretched thin without breaking. In case the dough cracks, it isn't ready yet. Continue kneading and gradually adding water until you reach the desired consistency. When the dough is ready, press the sides inward to form a ball and dust it with flour.

Cover with a kitchen towel and let aside to expand for about two hours.

In a saucepan over high heat, heat the oil until it is about 3-inches deep.

Take a handful of dough and stretch it to the size of a bread slice. The center should be thin and stretchy with no rips, but the borders should be thicker for the time being. Fry, turning once, until the edges are golden brown (for approximately 3-minutes).

Allow to drain on paper towels and cool to room temperature.

To coat, dip in the sugar vesssel or shake in a bag.

Warm it up and enjoy it!Prepare the pears while the cake is cooking or cooling. In a non-reactive saucepan, combine the water, port, sugar, cinnamon stick, and strips of zest and bring to a simmer over medium heat, stirring to dissolve the sugar. Pears should be peeled, quartered, and cored before being sliced into 8 portions. Reduce the heat under the saucepan to a low simmer, then add the pear pieces and poach for 15 to 20 minutes (do not stir, since the fruit will become rather delicate). The pears will be mushy but retain their form after cooking and will have developed a rich maroon color. Remove them from the poaching liquid. Allow to cool after straining. Serve the pears beside the cake, with a scoop of vanilla ice cream or a dollop of crème fraîche on the side. PUDDING WITH RICE

4 servings

100 g (312 oz/generous 12 cup) of ingredients 650 mL (22 fl oz/234 cups) rice pudding 12 unwaxed lemon zest, peeled and sliced into long strips water sprinkle of salt

12 tsp cinnamon

812 fl oz (1 cup) 250 ml 40 g whole milk (112 oz/scant 14 cup) the caster (superfine) 2 egg yolks, sugar

1 tablespoon butter (ground cinnamon) for serving

Directions

Cook, uncovered, for roughly thirty minutes, until most of the water has drained and the rice is just soft enough in a pot with the water, salt, strips of lemon zest, and cinnamon stick over a low heat.

Heat the milk and sugar in a separate pan after the rice has been cooking for 25 minutes.

In a mixing bowl, whisk the egg yolks until smooth and creamy.

After thirty minutes, reduce the heat under the rice to the lowest level possible and begin to integrate the hot milk-and-sugar mixture into the cooked rice by adding it gently and often, mixing after each addition, similar to risotto. When everything is combined, the rice should have the consistency of thick porridge. Extinguish the flame. To temper the yolks, add a tablespoon of the hot rice mixture to the beaten yolks and incorporate quickly. Then, while still in the pot but off the heat, slowly incorporate the egg-yolk mixture into the remaining rice, mixing quickly. Return the saucepan to a very low heat, add the butter, and simmer for three minutes, stirring constantly to avoid the egg in the bottom of the pan from overheating and splitting.

Serve warm or cold, with cinnamon sprinkled over top, in four serving dishes.

BISCUITS FROM A CAT'S TONGUE

This recipe makes around 20 biscuits.

75 g (212 oz) of ingredients 100 g soft salted butter (312 oz/scant 12 cup) the caster (superfine) 12 teaspoon vanilla extract sugar 2 beaten egg whites

312 oz/34 cup 100 g merely (all-purpose) to grease with flour and flavorless oil (optional)

Directions

Preheat the oven to 200°C (400°F/Gas 6) in advance.

Cream the butter and sugar together in a stand mixer equipped with a beater attachment until light and creamy, then add the vanilla extract and egg whites, mixing briefly to incorporate. Finally, fold in the flour with a metal spoon or a spatula, swiping a swiping motion through the mixture until just incorporated — don't over-mix. Make the biscuit mix by hand if you choose. Use a silicone baking pan to cook these cookies if you have one, since they stick quickly. If not, gently coat a large non-stick baking sheet with oil. Fill a piping bag with the biscuit mixture and pipe 6 2 cm (212 34 in) pieces of the mixture onto the sheet, allowing at least 5 cm (2 in) between each one from side to side and around 3 cm (114 in) from top to bottom, since the biscuits will spread out a lot in the oven. Place in the oven for 8–10 minutes, or until the edges of the biscuits are golden brown (the centres may remain fairly pale). Remove the biscuits from the oven and use a palette knife or spatula to draw them onto a wire rack or dish to cool and firm up while still hot.

In a vacuum container, the biscuits will last for many days.

6 Servings Sweet Rice Pudding

14 teaspoon salt 14 teaspoon kosher salt 14 teaspoon kosher salt 14 teaspoon kosher salt 2 c. liquid

1 cup Italian sticky rice, big chunks of raw lemon rind

1 cinnamon stick

four and a half cups full milk (14 cup used with the egg yolks) four beaten egg yolks

1 teaspoon vanilla extract

14 cup butter (distributed)

Directions

Combine the water and salt in a pan.

Bring to a boil, then add the rice and stir to combine.

Reduce the heat to low and continue to cook, stirring often, until the rice has absorbed the majority of the liquid (about twenty minutes). Allowing it to totally dry out will cause it to burn. In a large mixing bowl, combine the lemon rind, half of the butter, the cinnamon stick, and four cups of milk. Raise the temperature to medium-high. Allow to return to a boil, stirring often, and then reduce to a low burner. Check for any rice that has adhered to the pan's bottom. Cooking time is 20 minutes. Add the remaining butter and continue to stir while boiling for about ten minutes. In a small vessel, whisk together the eggs and 14 cup milk. Pour the egg mixture into the remaining ingredients and simmer for a few minutes more, until the mixture thickens.

Remove the pan from the heat and stir in the vanilla extract.

Remove the lemon rinds and cinnamon stick and discard.

Pour onto a serving dish and season with a pinch of cinnamon on top.

Serve cold or at room temperature at all times. Serve and have fun! Doughnuts de Portugal (serves 20)

1 tbsp yeast 1 tbsp sugar 1 tbs

6 eggs, room temperature at all times

a third of a cup of warm water, split into two 12 pound portions flour for baking

14 cup milk 12 teaspoon salt tablespoons vegetable shortening four tablespoons sugar, divided

a third of a cup of water, oil for frying, and sugar for sprinkling

Directions

In a 14 cup of warm water, dissolve your yeast and 1 teaspoon of sugar, then set away.

Beat your eggs with 1 spoonful of sugar in a vesssel until they achieve a thick consistency.

Melt the butter in a saucepan, then add the milk, shortening, and the remaining heated water. Allow to cool to a certain level.

While mixing, decant in the egg yolks.

Combine the flour and salt in a mixing bowl.

Pour in the egg mixture and mix with your fingertips.

Half of the water is added, and the mixture is folded in half from the edges to the middle. Repeat as needed.

Knead in your yeast mixture and continue to knead.

Gradually add additional water to the vesssel, making the dough moist and sticky.

Continue to knead the dough until it begins to stay together.

Take a portion the size of an egg and stretch it out to test whether it can be stretched thin without breaking. In case the dough cracks, it isn't ready yet. Continue kneading and gradually adding water until you reach the desired consistency. When the dough is ready, press the sides inward to form a ball and dust it with flour.

Cover with a kitchen towel and let aside to expand for about two hours.

In a saucepan over high heat, heat the oil until it is about 3-inches deep.

Take a handful of dough and stretch it to the size of a bread slice. The center should be thin and stretchy with no rips, but the borders should be thicker for the time being. Fry, turning once, until the edges are golden brown (for approximately 3-minutes).

Allow to drain on paper towels and cool to room temperature.

To coat, dip in the sugar vesssel or shake in a bag.

Warm it up and enjoy it!

Chapter 5

INCH ROUND BREADS

EANS, DRIED feijo (fay-zhowhn) for one to two hours, or until the bean water takes on the color of the black beans and appears muddy. Remove the beans from the heat as soon as they are tender enough.

IN ORDER TO MAKE THE GREENS

Combine the collard greens, salt, garlic, and 6 quarts water in a separate big saucepan. Bring the water to a boil over high heat. Reduce the heat to medium-low and continue to cook until the greens are tender, about thirty minutes. Remove the flame and set it aside.

Combine the bouillon, salt, and 6 cups water in a medium saucepan. Bring the water to a boil over high heat. Add the rice, stir, and bring to a boil once more. Reduce the heat to low, cover, and cook for 25 to 30 minutes, or until the rice is soft enough. Fluff the rice with a fork, cover, and set aside. Stir the beans and check the water's color. Remove the beans when the water starts to take on the color of the beans and they are soft enough. Divide the rice, collard greens, beans, pork and sausage, and the remaining orange slices among the serving dishes evenly. Pea and Chourico

4–6 SERVINGS

12 pound chouriço, peeled and sliced 1 medium yellow onion, quartered and sliced 2 minced garlic cloves

1 tbsp Pimenta de Moida

14 teaspoon all-spice blend from Portugal

12 tsp. kosher salt, plus more if necessary 2 pound peas (fresh or frozen)

3 tablespoons extra virgin olive oil lager beer, 12 oz.

12 CUP TOMATO SUGAR 4–6 eggs, large

Directions

Heat the olive oil in a big saucepan over medium heat. Cook for two minutes after adding the onion. Cook for three to four minutes with the chouriço and garlic, being careful not to overcook the garlic.

Mix in the Pimenta Moida, All Spice, and salt until everything is well combined.

Mix in the peas, beer, tomato sauce, and 2 quarts water until everything is well combined. Increase the heat to medium-high and bring to a boil. Reduce the heat to medium-low, stir, cover, and cook, stirring periodically, for 15 to 20 minutes, or until the time is cooked through. Provide 4 to 6 indentations in the peas with a big spoon to make space for the eggs to poach. Make an indentation in each egg with a light crack. Cover and continue to cook for another ten minutes. Season with salt to taste.

Serve immediately with crusty bread.

Soup with Greens

6 SERVINGS

Ingredients: 5 pounds peeled and diced starchy potatoes 12 pound collard greens, sliced into thin ribbons 1 medium onion, finely chopped 2 garlic cloves, smashed 1 teaspoon salt, plus more if required

12 pound peeled and thinly sliced hot or mild chouriço

12 teaspoon white pepper, freshly crushed

Directions

Combine the potatoes, onion, garlic, salt, and 8 quarts water in a 10-quart saucepan. Bring the water to a boil over high heat. Reduce the heat to low, cover, and continue to cook until the potatoes are fork tender, about 45 minutes, checking periodically and adding water as required to keep the potatoes submerged.

Carefully puree the potato mixture in an electric blender until it is completely smooth.

Add the collard greens, chouriço, white pepper, and enough water to halfway fill the saucepan. Bring the water to a boil over high heat. Reduce the heat to low and continue to cook until the greens are tender enough to eat, about thirty minutes. Season with salt to taste.

Warm the dish before serving.

6–8 SERVINGS BEAN STOUP INGREDIENTS

IN THE CASE OF BEANS

16 oz. dried white navy beans, rinsed and inspected for stones 1 medium diced onion

2 crushed and minced garlic cloves

16 oz. dried white navy beans, rinsed and inspected for stones

TO MAKE THE SOUP

12 pound peeled and sliced hot chouriço 5 to 6 medium peeled and diced potatoes

2 oz. pork fat or bacon (uncured) (optional) 1 tbsp Pimenta de Moida

salt kosher

white pepper, freshly crushed small-shell pasta (8 ounces) tomato sauce (4 oz.)

Directions

THE BEANS MUST BE MADE IN A DIFFERENT WAY THAN THEY

Toss the beans, onion, garlic, and 8 quarts water together in a 10-quart saucepan. Bring to a boil over a high heat. Reduce to a low heat, cover, and simmer for 112 to 2 hours, or until the beans are soft enough. Check the beans often and, if necessary, add just enough water to cover them.

-

SOUP PREPARE

Fill the kettle halfway with water. In a large mixing bowl, combine the chouriço, potatoes, pig fat (if using), Pimenta Moida, a good amount of salt, and the white pepper. Allow to come to a boil over medium-high heat.

Reduce the heat to medium-low, cover, and simmer, stirring often, for around thirty minutes, or until the potatoes are soft enough.

Cook, stirring often, for thirty minutes, with the pasta.

Blend in the tomato sauce. Taste and season with salt if necessary. Warm food is best.

Refrigerate leftovers for up to five days in a vacuum jar.

BREADS

CORN BREAD\sMAKES 2 ROUND LOAVES

Ingredients\s2 packages active dry yeast 1 cup warm water (110°f)

3½ cups unbleached bread flour, plus more for dusting 2 cups fine yellow cornmeal (preferably goya brand) (preferably goya brand)

2 tablespoons kosher salt 1¼ cups boiling water

Coarse cornmeal, for dusting

Directions

Dissolve the yeast in the warm water in a small vesssel and let stand till the time the liquid is foamy, approximately ten minutes. Stir in 1½ cups of the bread flour, cover with plastic wrap, and add in a warm spot till the time doubled in size, approximately forty- five minutes. Dump the fine cornmeal and salt into the vesssel of a stand blender fitted with the paddle attachment. Decant in the boiling water and blend on medium speed till the time a firm dough clumps together, approximately three minutes. Let sit till the time the yeast blend is done. Switch to the mixer's dough hook, scoop in the remainder of the 2 cups of bread flour and the yeast blend, and knead on low, adding more flour, a bit at a time in case needed, till the time the blend comes together into a firm, elastic dough that cleans the sides of the vesssel, approximately 7 minutes. Line a 13-by-18-inch rimmed baking sheet with parchment and drizzle with coarse cornmeal; put aside. Turn the dough out onto a lightly floured surface and knead not many times. In case the dough is sticking, drizzle with a bit of flour. Cut it in half and shape each piece into a ball. Cup one ball in both hands and stretch the sides of the dough down and under, making an oval, then turn 90 degrees and repconsume, crconsuming a smooth round with a tight surface. Securely pinch the seams closed underneath and turn seam side down. Replicate with the second ball of dough. Dust the loaves heavily with bread flour. Transfer to the baking sheet, cover with a tea towel, and let rise in a warm, draft-free spot till the time doubled in size, approximately forty-five minutes. Position a rack in the centre of the oven. Put a heavy-bottomed skillet on the floor of the oven, and crank up the heat to 475°F. Uncover the loaves and Take the baking sheet into the oven, then lean back and decant 1½ cups of water into the skillet. Close the door swiftly. (The steam will make a lovely crunchy crust.) Wait for five minutes, and repeat. Bake till the time the loaves are golden brown and crackly—charred in spots isn't a bad thing—and sound hollow when thwacked on the bottom, 35 to forty-five minutes. Transfer to a rack to cool till the time just warm. These are best devoured the same day.

MADEIRAN GRIDDLE BREAD\sMAKES SIX 6-

Ingredients\s1 small sweet potato (about 5 ounces) (about 5 ounces)

1 tablespoon plus 1 teaspoon active dry yeast 1 teaspoon plus 1 tablespoon sugar

1¼ cups warm water (110°f)

3¼ cups all-purpose flour, plus more in case needed 1¾ teaspoons kosher salt\stablespoon unsalted butter, always at room temperature Olive oil\sroasted garlic butter with madeira, always at room temperature

Directions

Prick the sweet potato wholly over with a fork, pop it into the microwave, and zap on high till the time softened, approximately five minutes. As another option, transfer the potato on a foil-lined baking sheet and roast in a 400°F oven till the time soft, approximately 40 minutes. The moment the potato is optimally cool to handle, split it open and lift out the flesh, and toss out the peel. You must have access to about ½ cup. Let cool completely. Dissolve the yeast and the 1 teaspoon of sugar in ¼ cup of the warm water in a small vesssel and let stand till the time the liquid is foamy, approximately ten minutes. Meld the potato, flour, the remainder of the 1 tablespoon of sugar, and the salt in an electronic blender. Whir till the time the potato is pulverized and no lumps remain. Put in the butter and the yeast blend and pulse till the time incorporated. With the motor running, decant in the remainder of the 1 cup of warm water and buzz till the time the dough just forms a smooth ball that springs back a bit when poked, 30 to 45 seconds. Add more flour a bit at a time in case needed. Lightly coat a big vesssel with oil. Dump the dough onto a work surface, shape it into a ball, set it in the vesssel, and turn to coat. Cover the vesssel with plastic wrap, place it in a warm, draft-free spot, and let the dough double in size, approximately 1½ hours. Spread a tea towel on a work surface and lightly dust it and the work surface Now to it with flour. Plop out the dough and cut it into six equal pieces. Roll each piece into a ball with your palm, press it down to a thickness of ¾ inch, and Set on the tea towel. Cover with another tea towel and let stand till the time puffed considerably, 30 to forty-five minutes.

Position a rack in the centre of the oven and crank up the heat to 350°F.

Warm a flat griddle or a large heavy nonstick skillet over medium-high flame for five minutes. Slip one hand under the towel, turn a dough circle onto your other hand, and slide it onto the griddle. Cook, pushing down lightly with a spatula to make a golden- brown underside, approximately four minutes. Flip and brown the second side for 2 to

three minutes. Slip the bolo onto a baking sheet and replicate with the remainder of the circles of dough. Take the baking sheet into the oven and bake the breads till the time cooked through, approximately fifteen minutes. Transfer to a rack and cool for not many minutes. Slice the breads horizontally in half and generously slather with the garlic butter. Slice into strips and serve immediately.

BERLIM CUSTARD DOUGHNUTS

Turn the pastry rectangle so 1 of the long sides is facing you. Lightly roll it out to make

a square again, being careful not to burst the layers of butter when you reach the edges of the pastry. Replicate the spreading-folding process with the second third of the butter, with the help of lots of flour on the work surface and rolling pin again. Chill again in case needed. To utilize the final third of the butter, roll out the pastry into a rectangle coarsely 45 × 55 cm (18 × 22 in), with the help of lots of flour under the pastry and on the rolling pin. Working swiftly, spread the remainder of the butter wholly over the pastry, leaving a 3 cm (1¼ in) gap around the edge. Spread it as thinly as you can, nonetheless be gentle, as the pastry will be fragile and prone to tearing. Starting with a shorter edge, roll the pastry into a tight Swiss roll or log shape, strokeing off extra flour as you proceed. Trim the ends so that the edges are even, Slice the log in half, wrap the two halves in plastic wrap and chill in the refrigerator at the very least 3 hours or for nightlong. (You can freeze all or half of the pastry at this stage. Defrost for nightlong in the refrigerator before using.) in case using half the pastry, to make 12 tarts, remember to make half the quantity of custard. To make the custard, transfer the sugar and water in a saucepan and heat till the time the blend reaches 105°C (221°F) on a saucepan thermometer. Put the flame out and set it aside. In a different pan, heat the milk till the time just below boiling point, then put in the vanilla pod, cinnamon stick and lemon rind. Take off of the flame and let rest to infutilize for five minutes or so.

Meld and mix the egg yolks in a large heavy vesssel till the time smooth and creamy.

Take out the vanilla pod, cinnamon and lemon rind from the milk. Skim off any skin which has formed. Add a tablespoon of the hot milk to the egg yolks and whisk vigorously. Continue adding the hot milk, a tablespoon at a time, adding it slowly nonetheless whisking swiftly, so that the eggs don't cook and scramble. After adding 6–7 tablespoons of milk, slowly decant the remainder of the hot milk into the vesssel, continually beating the blend. Lastly, put in the sugar syrup in a stable stream, whisking uninterruptedly. Swiftly wash the milk pan, then transfer the custard blend back into it. Place the saucepan over the lowest possible heat and cook the custard very, very lightly, mixing uninterruptedly and running a spatula around the bottom and edges of the saucepan every now and then, to make certain all the liquid is moving all the time. After 8–25 minutes of gentle cooking, reliant on your pan, the blend should commence to thicken. In case you have access to access to a saucepan thermometer, thickening will occur at approximately 75°C (167°F). Don't allow to get hotter than 80°C (176°F) as the custard may split. The moment the custard has thickened to the consistency of double cream, take out it from the heat and decant into a clean, heat resistant vesssel. Cover the surface with plastic wrap to prevent a skin forming, and put aside.

An hour before you want to cook the tarts, heat beforehand your oven to its maximum

temperature, ideally 275°C (525°F/Gas 10). In case you have access to access to a pizza stone, place it on the top shelf of the oven, or utilize a baking tray. Put a second pizza stone, or another baking tray, on the centre shelf of the oven. Let them both get really hot. This is the best method to replicate the fierce heat of bakery ovens, and will allow the tarts to cook swiftly with crunchy bases and (hopefully) to caramelise on top. Leave optimum space between the stones or trays for the tarts. Now, grease the holes of a shallow 12-hole tart tin (of the sort you'd make jam tarts in, instead of muffins). Take out 1 of the pastry logs from the refrigerator and leave it for approximately ten minutes till the time it becomes pliable. Slice it into 12 discs and place each one, cut side down, into the tin. Have ready a cup of chilled water. Dip your thumbs into the water and lightly press the dough downwards and outwards, pushing it into the edges of the tin and upwards and outwards so that, at last, it fans out approximately 1 cm (½ in) above the side of the tin. Try not to pinch these protruding edges though – in case you can leave them a bit of thicker, they will frill out during cooking.

The pastry will be approximately 2 mm (⅛ in) thick at this point. Press the pastry edges to some extent outwards, so that they don't collapse inwards as they cook. They should be in the shape of an inverted hat with a brim. Decant the custard into each tart case, filling them generously and leaving approximately 7.5 mm (¼ in) of the pastry rim showing. Cautiously Take the tray into the very hot oven. Bake the tarts for 10–1six minutes, possibly to some extent longer in case your oven can't reach very high temperatures, checking them every few minutes after the first ten minutes.

The pastry edges may shrink down to some extent and may appear to overcook a bit of, nonetheless hold your nerve: to some extent burnt bitterness is part of their characteristic flavour, and in case you take them out from the oven as well soon, the custard won't caramelise on top. (I have to admit that caramelising the custard remains a bit of a dark art – every now and then it happens and every now and then it doesn't. You can utilize a blowtorch in case you really want, nonetheless your pasteis de nata will appear more like crème brûlées.) When prepared, the tart pastry will be brown and occasionally even to some extent charred, with not many brown spots on top of the custard. Take out and leave the tarts to cool in the tin. (Don't worry in case a bit of butter appears to have escaped from the pastry – as they cool, this will resolve itself.)

Clean the tin and replicate with the second half of the pastry, in case using.

Eat warm, sprinkled with a bit of icing sugar and ground cinnamon.

SANTA CLARA PASTRIES Makes 6 pastries

Ingredients four egg yolks

125 g (four oz/½ cup) caster (superfine) (superfine) sugar 75 ml (2½ fl oz/ cup) water

couple of drops of freshly squeezed lemon juice

75 g (2½ oz/¾ cup) ground almonds (almond meal) 100 g (3½ oz) butter, melted 6 sheets of filo pastry, measuring coarsely 20 × 30 cm (8 × 12 in) icing (confectioners') sugar for dusting

Directions

Meld and mix the egg yolks in a heavy mixing vesssel till the time smooth and creamy.

Put a deep saucepan over a high flame and put in the sugar, water and lemon juice. Heat the blend till the time it reaches 105°C (221°F) on a saucepan thermometer. Take off of the flame and let cool for a number of minutes. Decant the syrup, very slowly, over the egg yolks, beating uninterruptedly with a whisk. Once all the syrup has been added to the yolks, decant the blend back into the pan. Place over a very low flame and cook, mixing, for five-ten minutes, or till the time the blend thickens – it should appear like a bright yellow or orange custard. (Don't let the blend get as well hot, or boil, as the yolks will scramble.) Take off of the flame and stir in the ground almonds. Put aside to cool a bit of. Heat beforehand the oven to 200°C (400°F/Gas 6) and grease a baking sheet with a bit of the melted butter. When working with filo, Place the unutilized sheets under a clean damp tea towel, as filo dries out and becomes brittle very swiftly. Put down one sheet of filo on a work surface. Cut it into 2 rectangles. Stroke one rectangle with melted butter, then transfer the other rectangle on top. Stroke with melted butter again. Spread a generous tablespoon of the almond filling on top of the pastry, a third of the way from the base of the pastry, and halfway from the sides. (Don't overfill as the pastries may burst in the oven.) Turn the bottom side in, covering the filling, then fold twice more to enfold the filling. Position the now to some extent flattened pastry tube so that the seam is on the bottom. Press gently on the fold on either side of the filling, pushing the filling so it sits the middle of the tube with a gap on either side – this creates space within the pastry for the filling to expand during cooking. Stroke the top of the pastry with butter. Lightly pinch each of the ends of the tube together, then fold inwards. Stroke the newly exposed pastry with butter. Set on the

baking sheet and continue with the remaining filo and filling to make 6 pastries.

Bake in the oven for 12–1three minutes, till the time the pastry is golden and crisp.

Take out the pastries from the oven, allow them to cool to some extent, then dust with icing sugar. Serve warm or always at room temperature. EGG THREADS

Serves 4

Ingredients 8 egg yolks

300 g (10 ½ oz/1½ cups) caster (superfine) (superfine) sugar
200 ml (7 fl oz/generous ¾ cup) water

Directions

Transfer the yolks in a sieve as you separate them, to take out as much white as possible, then transfer them to a vesssel. Beat the yolks together for a short time, so the egg is smooth, nonetheless without introducing as well much air as this can make the threads puffy. Decant the yolks into a piping bag with a narrow nozzle attached, or into a plastic sandwich bag. Put aside. In the meantime, transfer the sugar and water in a wide frying saucepan and allow to come to a boil over a medium–high flame. Cook till the time to some extent thickened nonetheless not yet turning brown or caramelising (you want a thin, clear syrup), then turn down the flame till the time barely simmering.

Have ready a vesssel of iced water.

When prepared to cook, in case using a plastic sandwich bag, snip a 2 mm (⅛ in) hole in the corner of the bag. Sprinkle the yolk blend into the syrup, working from one side of the saucepan to the other and using a smooth back-and-forth motion to make long, thin threads in the syrup. Cook for thirty seconds, then lift out lightly, using a slotted spoon. Transfer the threads in the vesssel of iced water, trying to avoid tangling them.

Continue till the time all the yolks have been utilized up.

Serve as they are, in small vesssel, or utilize the threads to embellish cakes or confectionary.

MILK TARTS

Makes 12 tarts

Ingredients 500 ml (17 fl oz/2¼ cups) whole milk 25 g (1 oz) salted butter 100 g (3½ oz/¾ cup) plain (all-purpose) flour, plus more to dust 250 g (9 oz/1¼ cups) caster (superfine) (superfine) sugar

four eggs grated zest of ½ unwaxed lemon

½ teaspoon vanilla extract icing (confectioners') sugar, in order to serve ground cinnamon, in order to serve

Directions

Grease 12 paper cupcake cases and dust with flour. Heat beforehand the oven to 200°C (400°F/Gas 6). Heat the milk in a saucepan over medium flame till the time just below boiling point, then take off of the flame and put in the butter. Stir till the time the butter is entirely melted. Meld the flour and sugar in a vesssel, put in the eggs, lemon zest and vanilla extract, then beat just till the time smooth. Now, decant in the hot milk–butter blend in a stable stream while uninterruptedly whisking the batter. Using a ladle or jug, divide the batter, which will be very thin, uniformly between the cases. Add in the oven and cook for 25–35 minutes, till the time nicely browned on top and puffed up. Take off of the oven and let rest to cool in the cases – they will collapse nonetheless don't worry, that's what they do. The moment they're optimally cool to handle, transfer to a wire rack. Serve warm or always at room temperature, sprinkled with a bit of icing sugar and cinnamon. BREAD OF GOD

Makes 12 rolls

Ingredients BREAD

1 tablespoon active dry yeast 200 ml (8½ fl oz/1 cup) to some extent warm whole milk 50 g (2 oz/¼ cup) caster (superfine) (superfine) sugar four cm (1½ in) fragment of vanilla pod, split lengthways 1 egg, beaten 500 g (1 lb 2 oz/four cups) plain (all-purpose) flour, plus more to dust

½ teaspoon fine salt

four tablespoons salted butter, melted and cooled to some extent

TOPPING 2 eggs, beaten 125 g (four oz/½ cup) caster (superfine) (superfine) sugar 125 g (four oz) desiccated coconut icing (confectioners') sugar, to dust

Directions

Activate the yeast by mixing it in a jug or vesssel with the just-warm milk and sugar. Leave for ten minutes – it should develop a frothy head. Scrape the seeds out of the vanilla pod and meld and mix them into the yeast blend accompanied by the egg. Transfer the flour into a large mixing vesssel, put in the salt and the cooled melted butter, then put in the yeast blend. Mix to blend and, once it has formed a rough, sticky dough, turn onto a clean floured work surface and knead with the help of floured hands, for approximately ten minutes. As another option, utilize a stand blender fitted with a dough hook and knead for five minutes instead. The moment the dough is soft, stretchy and elastic, transfer it into a lightly oiled vesssel, cover with plastic wrap, and leave it in a warm place to rise for one hour or more, till the time doubled in size. Once the dough has risen, knock it back lightly, with the help of your knuckles to squash it back to more or less its original size. Divide into 12 equal-sized pieces and roll each one into a neat ball. Set on a large baking sheet sprinkled with flour, then cover with a clean tea towel and let rest to rise in a warm place for another thirty minutes. When prepared to cook, heat beforehand the oven to 175°C (340°F/Gas 3½). Lightly stroke the tops of each bread with beaten egg. Then mix the rest of the beaten egg into the sugar and coconut, to make a thick paste. Top each bread with a generous couple of spoonfuls of the topping, with the help of your hands to shape it so that it sits fairly flat on top of the breads. Add in the oven and cook for twenty minutes, till the time the breads are light gold and speckled with brown flecks. Take off of the oven and let rest to cool for ten minutes, then dust with icing sugar and Consume warm with a cup of coffee. FRESH CHEESE WITH HONEY & ALMONDS Serves 4

Ingredients four heaped tablespoons flaked almonds

1 × 200 g (7 oz) Queijo Fresco Cheese, always at room temperature four teaspoons good-quality honey

Directions

Lightly toast the almonds in a dry frying saucepan over a low flame till the time they turn a light golden brown.

Divide the cheese between four plates. Spread over the toasted almonds and sprinkle with the honey. Serve instantly.
MOLOTOV PUDDING

Makes 6 puddings

Ingredients flavourless oil, to grease

four fresh egg whites, always at room temperature pinch of fine salt

four tablespoons caster (superfine) sugar, plus 100 g (3½ oz/scant ½ cup)

½ teaspoon vanilla extract

3 tablespoons flaked or slivered almonds, in order to serve

Directions

With the help of vegetable oil on a fragment of paper towel, lightly grease 6 × 150 ml (5 fl oz/ ⅔ cup) individual pudding moulds.

Heat beforehand the oven to 180°C (350°F/Gas 4). Boil the kettle. Meld and mix the egg whites in a spotlessly clean vesssel with the salt till the time they form soft peaks. Put in the four tablespoons of sugar gradually, whisking uninterruptedly, then put in the vanilla extract and whisk for 4–5 minutes, or till the time the egg whites are smooth, shimmering and very thick. Spoon the blend into the pudding moulds, using a teaspoon to lightly force the blend into the corners of the mould. Smooth the tops and tap each mould lightly on the counter, to dislodge any big bubbles. Transfer the moulds in a large baking dish and fill it with boiling water till the time the water reaches halfway up the moulds. Transfer the tray in the oven and cook for 12 minutes. The puddings will brown a bit of and puff up mightily, nonetheless will deflate once you take them out from the oven. Take off of the water bath and let rest to cool in their tins, then lightly un-mould and transfer the puddings browned- side down on 6 dessert plates.

Toast the almonds lightly in a dry frying saucepan over a low flame. Put aside. In case you are serving this with the water caramel, boil the remainder of the sugar in a saucepan with 100 ml (3½ fl oz/scant ½ cup) water. Place the heat fairly high and boil hard. After a while, you will notice that the syrup gradually browns. Watch it like a hawk and Take off of the flame when it is still golden. Let cool for one to two minutes and check the consistency – it should be fairly watery so that you can drench the puddings with it. In case not, add some water, a tablespoon at a time, till the time it is thin sufficient, nonetheless be careful as it will bubble up as you do so. Serve the puddings always at room temperature with either the doce de leite, or this caramel sauce and maybe some custard, with the toasted almonds sprinkled on top. DULCE DE LECHE

Makes approximately 2 × 400 g (14 oz) jars

Ingredients 3 × 400 g (14 oz) tins sweetened condensed milk generous pinch of salt

Directions

Heat beforehand the oven to 220°C (425°F/Gas 7). Sterilise 2 heat resistant jars (including their lids) by cleaning them in hot soapy water, then transfer them in a low oven for fifteen minutes. Blend combining the condensed milk and salt in a glass or ceramic dish. Firmly cover the dish with foil. Set this dish inside a larger baking dish or tin, and fill it with hot water, till the time the water reaches just over halfway up the sides of the smaller dish. Add in the oven for one hour, keeping an eye on the water level and topping it up with more water from the kettle as necessary. After one hour, begin checking the colour of the milk – you are looking for a light golden brown colour to develop. Watch the water levels cautiously at this point; in case the water levels drop, then the milk will commence to bake and may take on a curdled, clotted appearance. The same will happen in case the foil comes loose. (In case the milk does seem to have split, don't panic. After taking the saucepan out of the oven, let cool just to some extent, then decant the split caramel into a big vesssel, leaving any over- browned, stuck-on milk in the original dish. Wearing oven gloves and long sleeves, cautiously beat the split blend with a heat resistant whisk, till the time fairly smooth. Now, set a sieve over another big vesssel, and strain out any rest of the lumps. The resulting sauce may have access to a very, very to some extent granular appearance, nonetheless it is so scrumptious, no one will notice.) Once the caramel is an even golden colour, cautiously Take off of the oven and let rest to cool a bit of. To preserve the caramel, while still hot, decant it into the clean, sterilised jars. Seal, cool, and keep in the refrigerator for up to 1 month.

CPSIA information can be obtained
at www.ICGtesting.com
Printed in the USA
LVHW061950240322
714086LV00009B/1072

9 781804 381212